I0791444

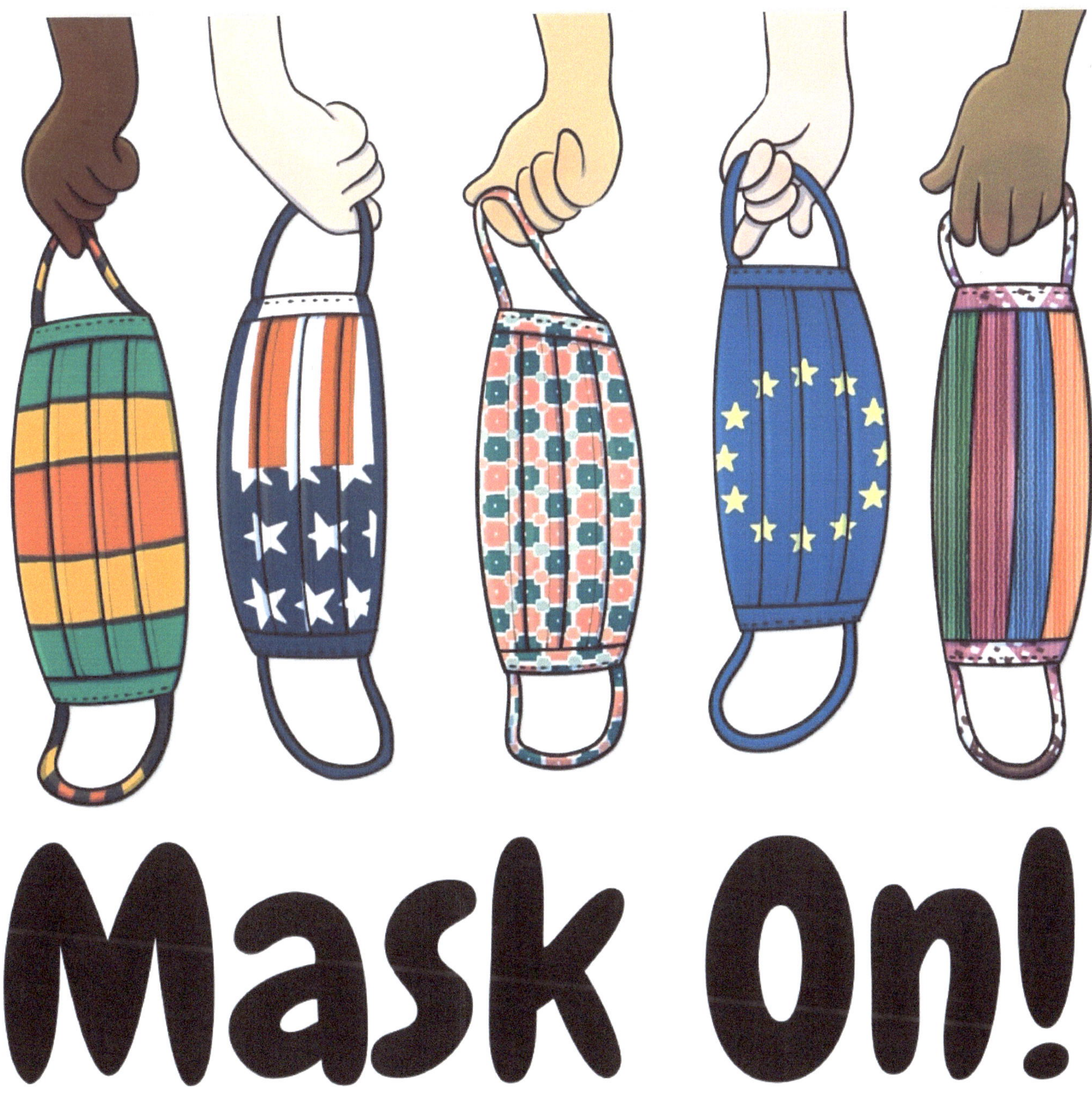

Mask On!

by **Tanisha Praise Mkandawire** *illustrated by* **"Muhammad At-Tayieb" Al-Hyari**

To Zion B. and all the little humans with
adventure on their minds and a BIG imagination.

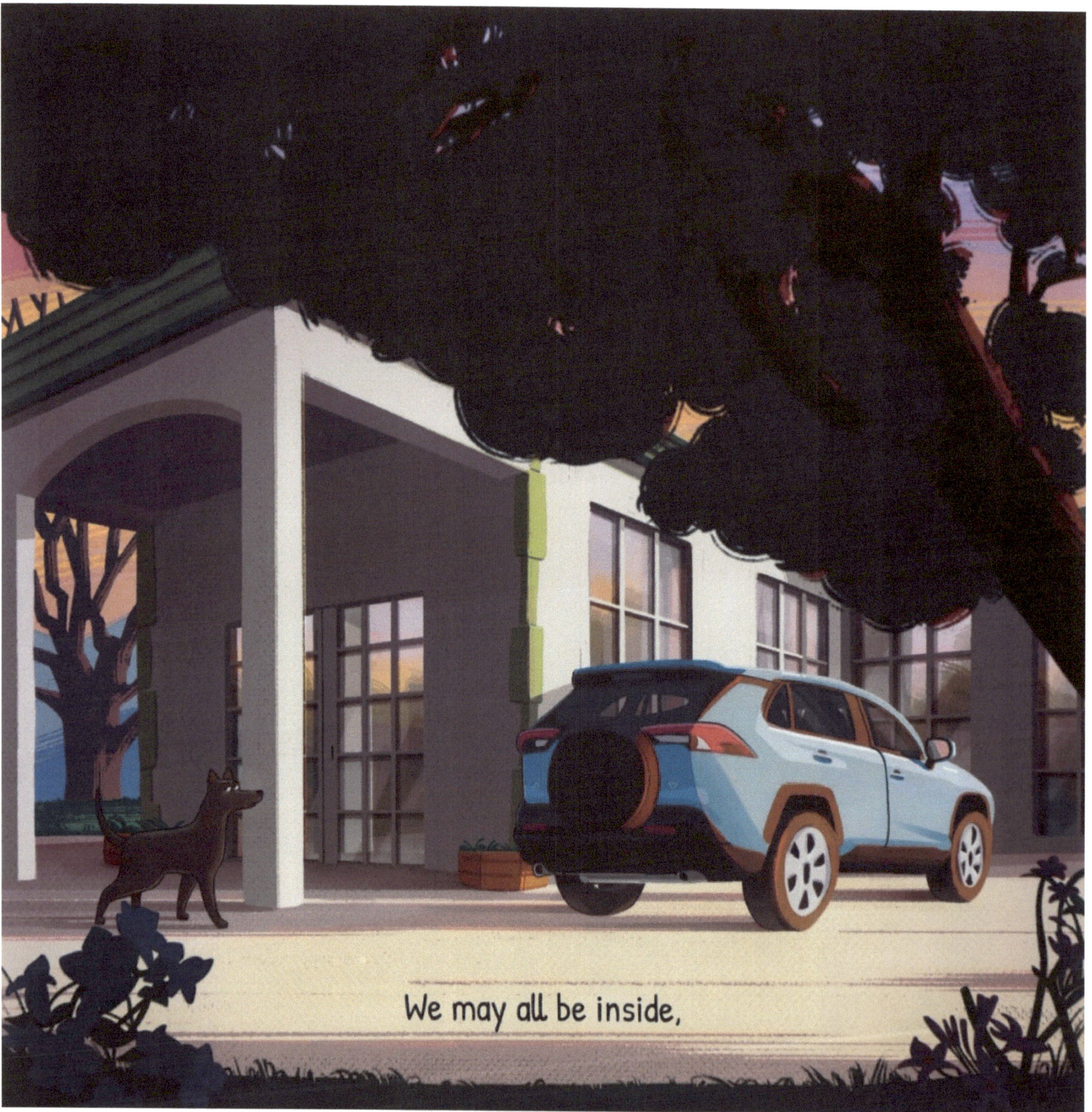

We may all be inside,

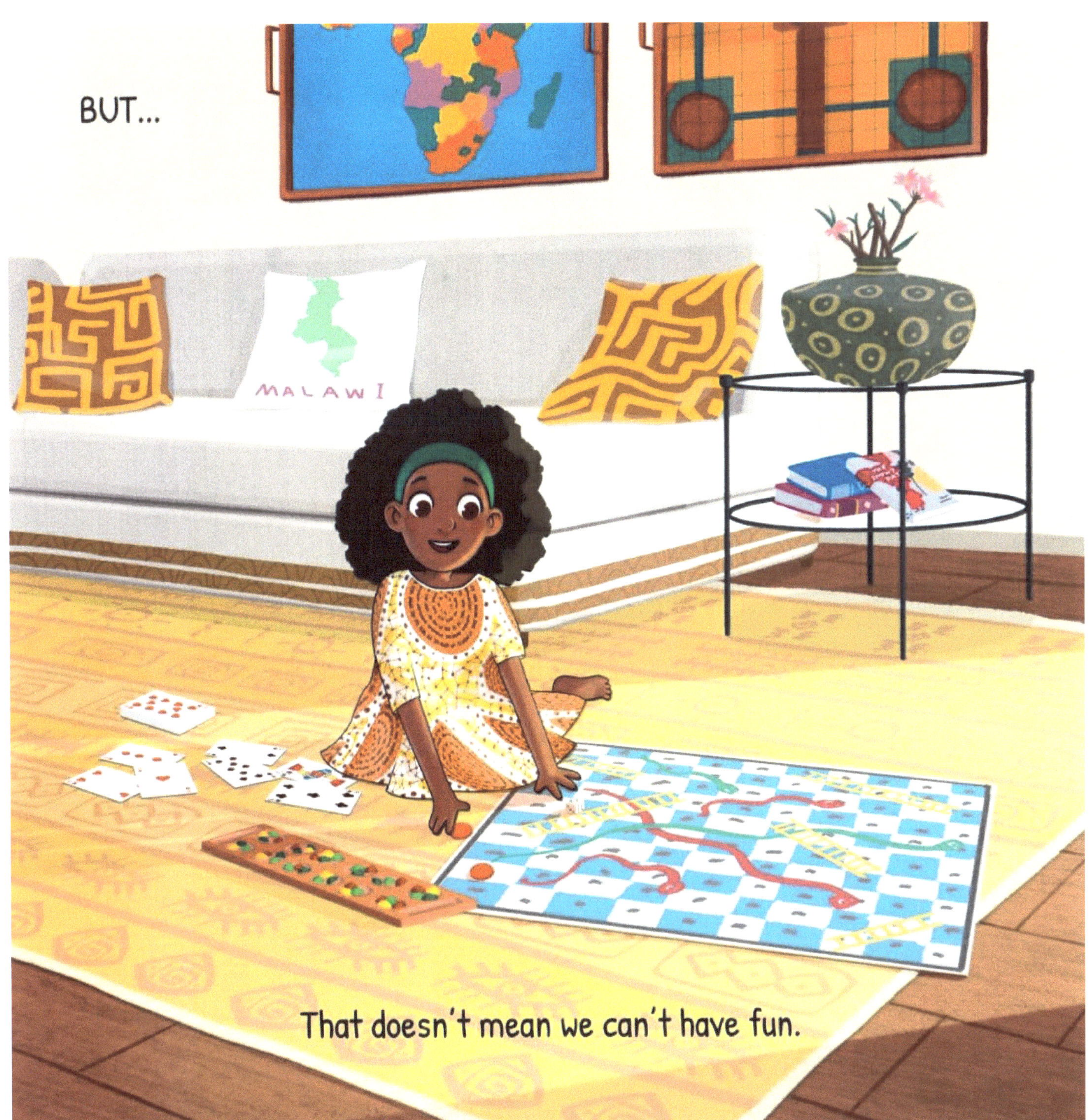
BUT...
MALAWI
That doesn't mean we can't have fun.

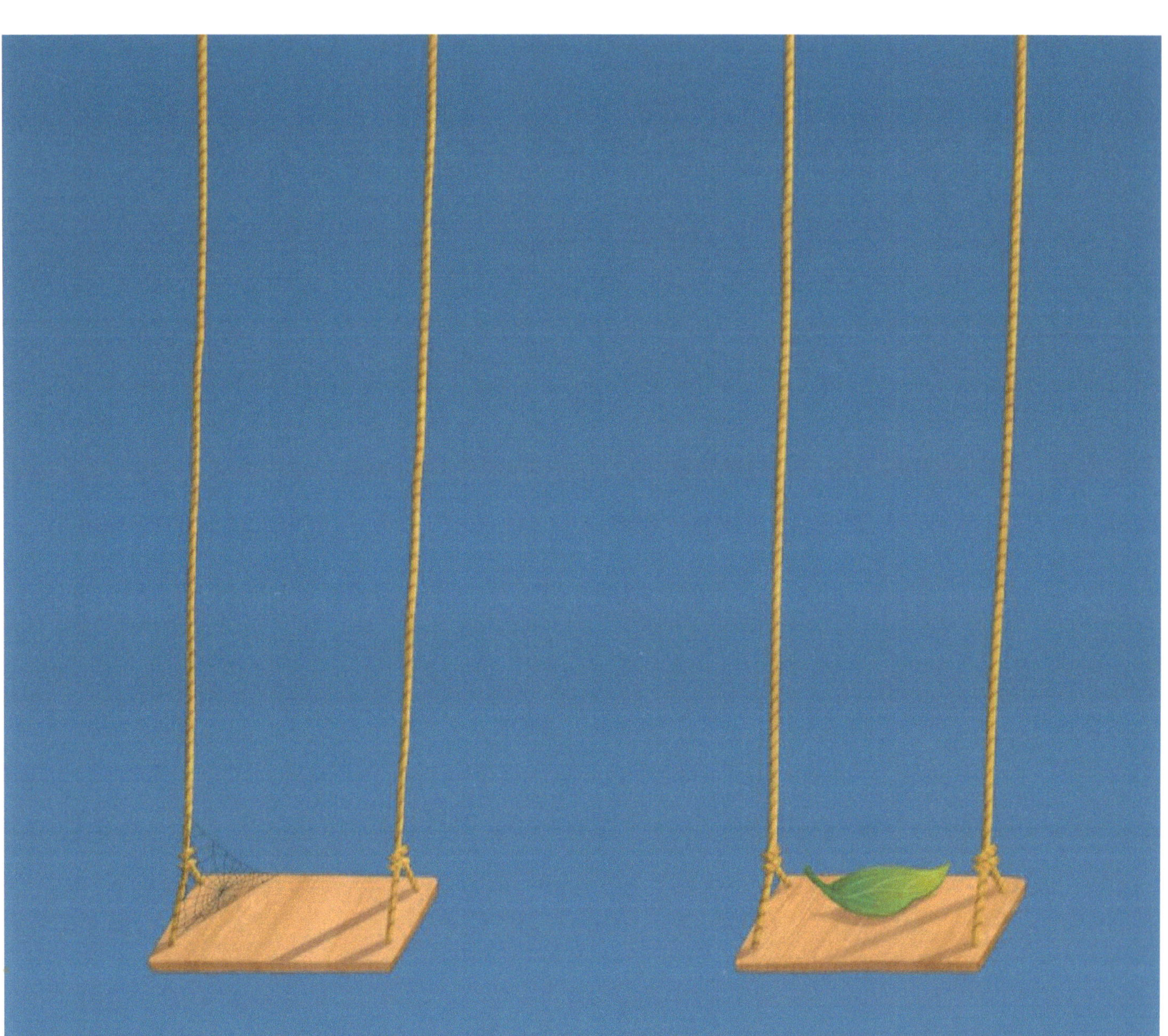

The playground may be closed,

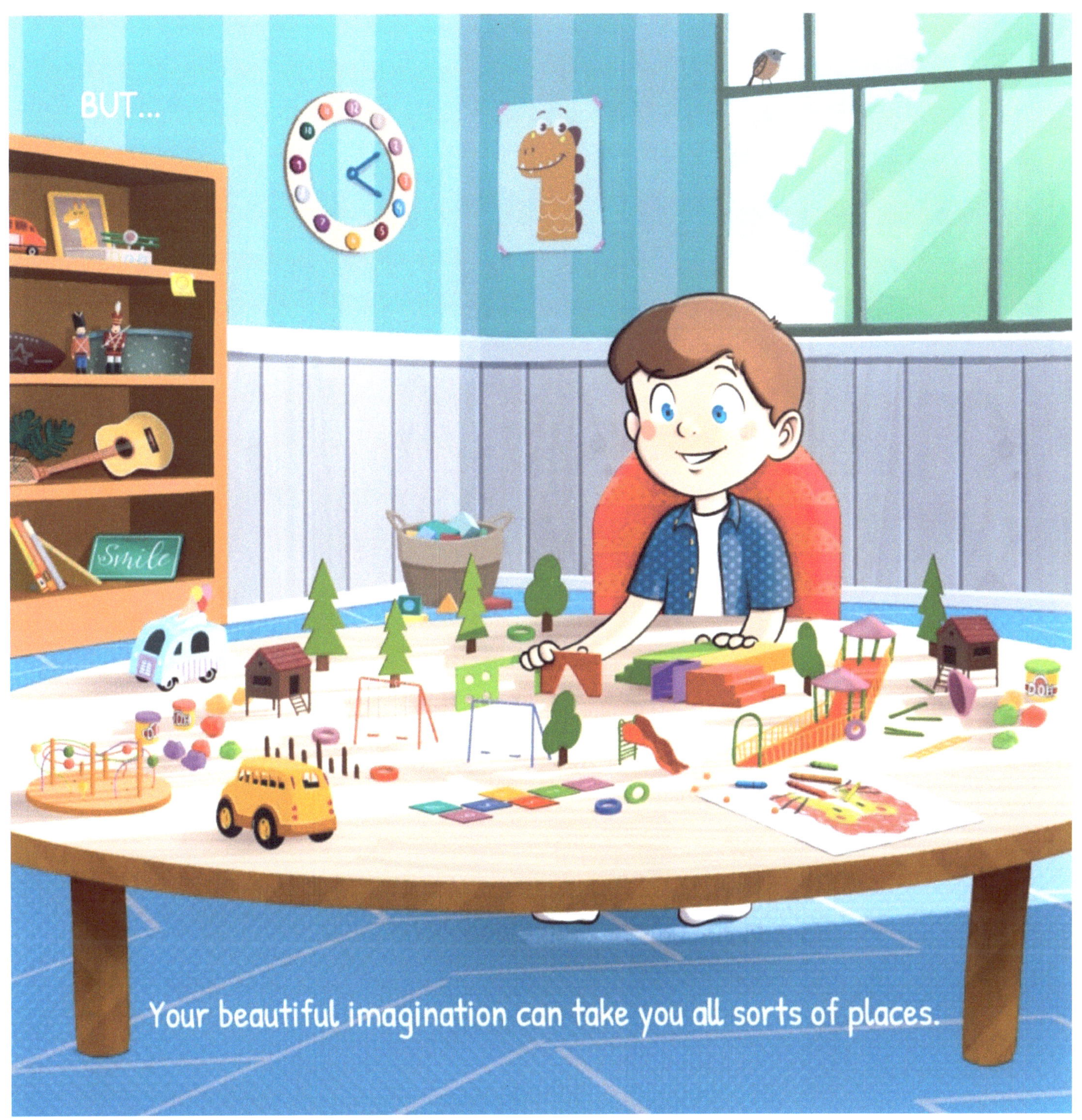

BUT...
Your beautiful imagination can take you all sorts of places.

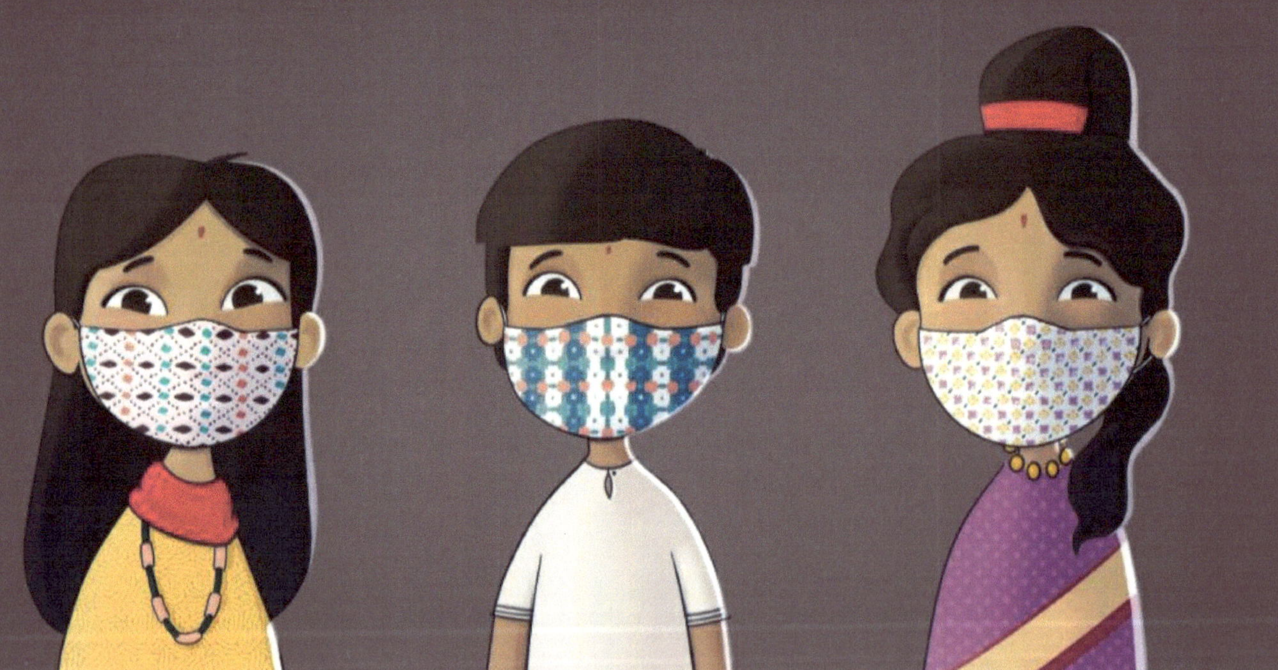

We might not be able to see your BIG smile,

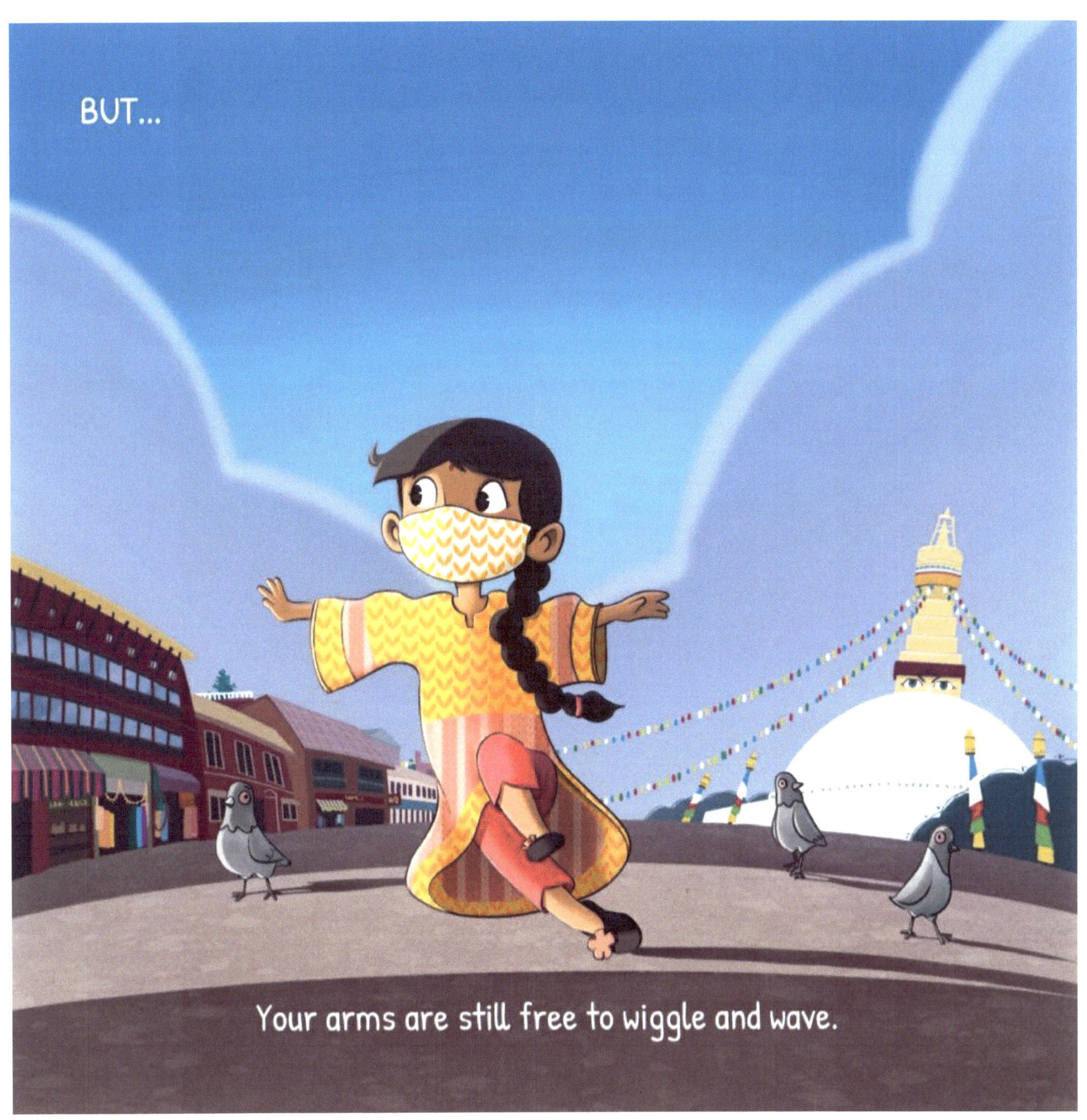

BUT...
Your arms are still free to wiggle and wave.

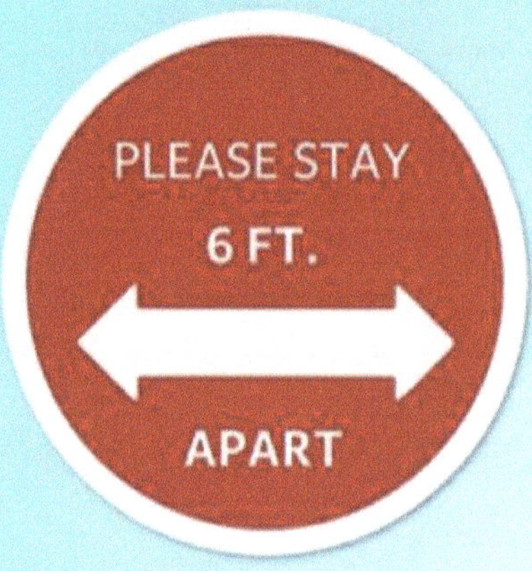

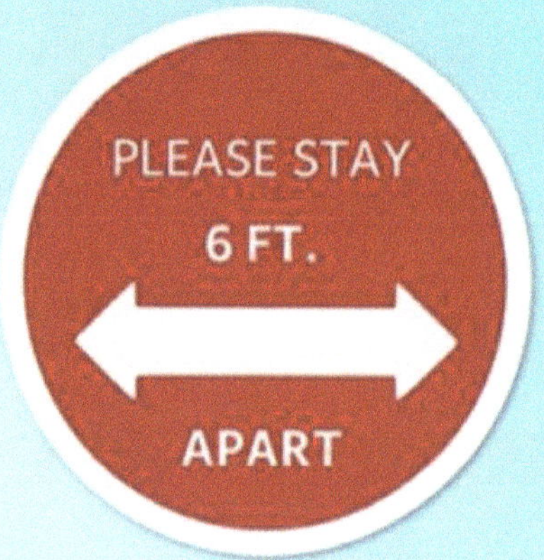

We have to stand 6ft apart,

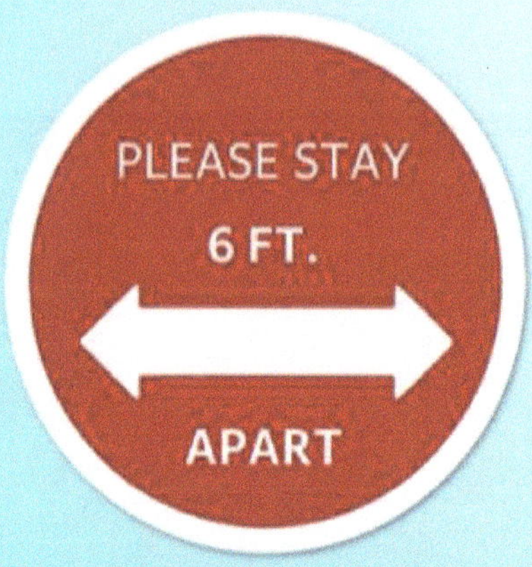

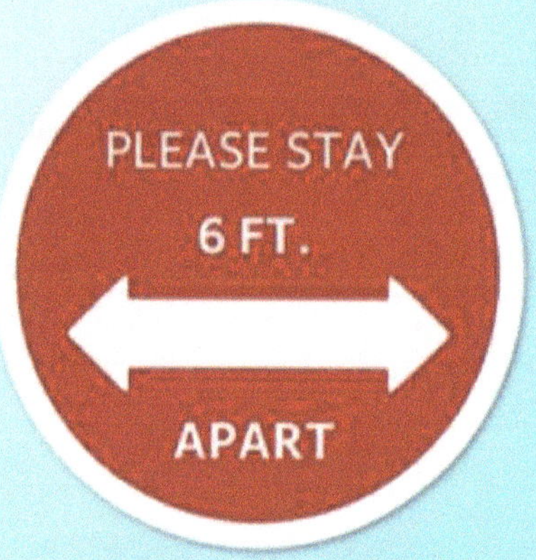

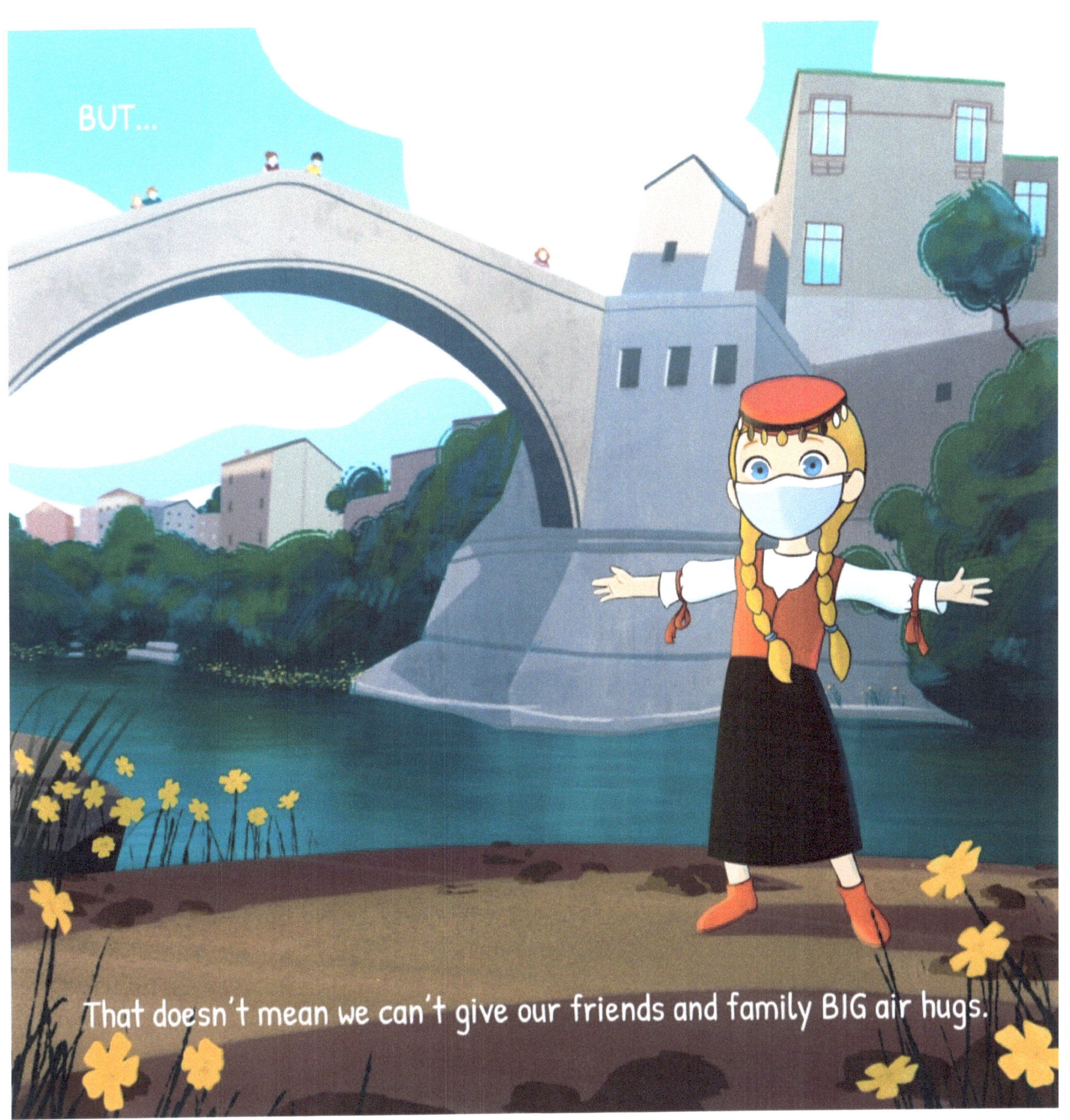

BUT...
That doesn't mean we can't give our friends and family BIG air hugs.

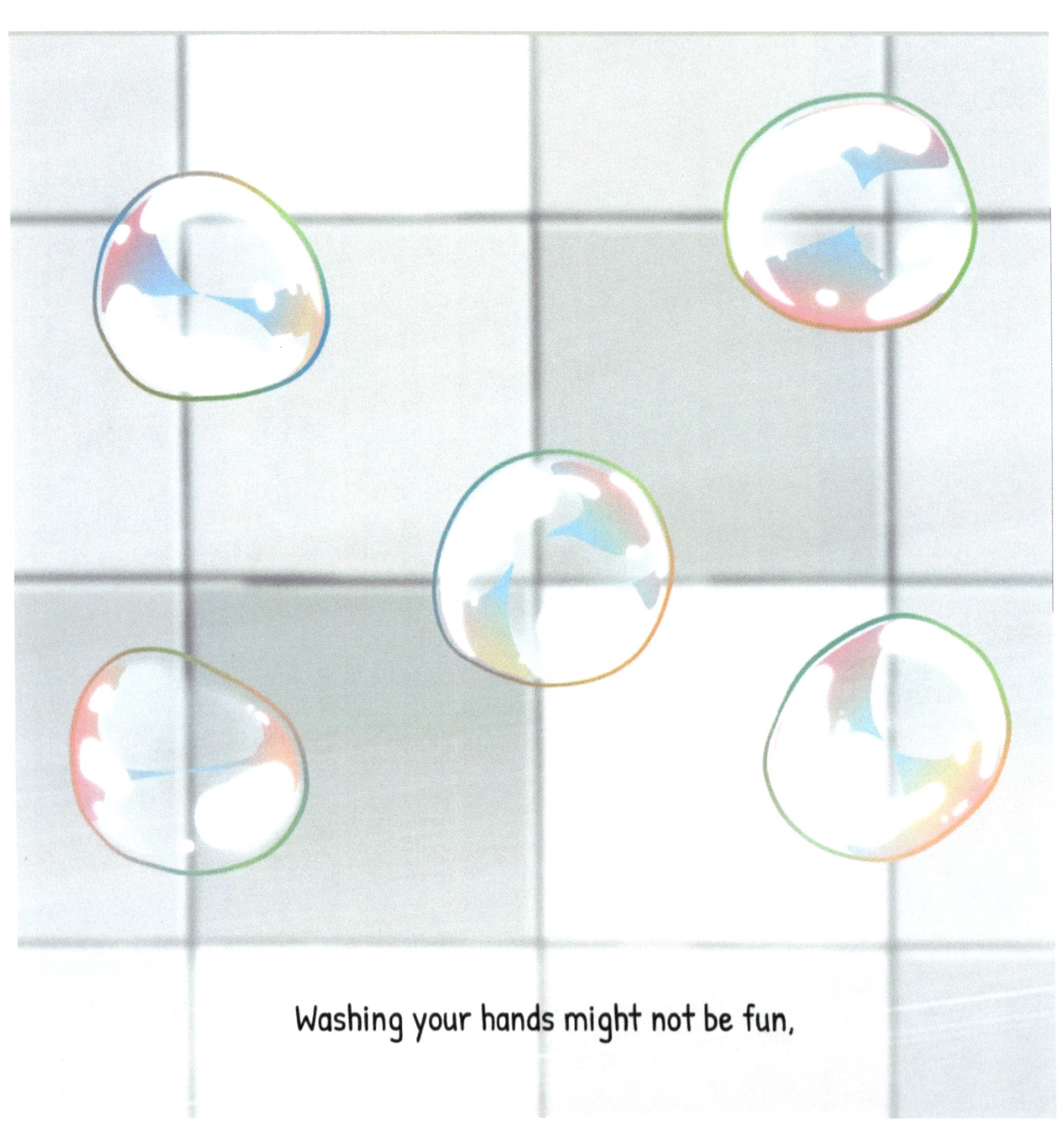

Washing your hands might not be fun,

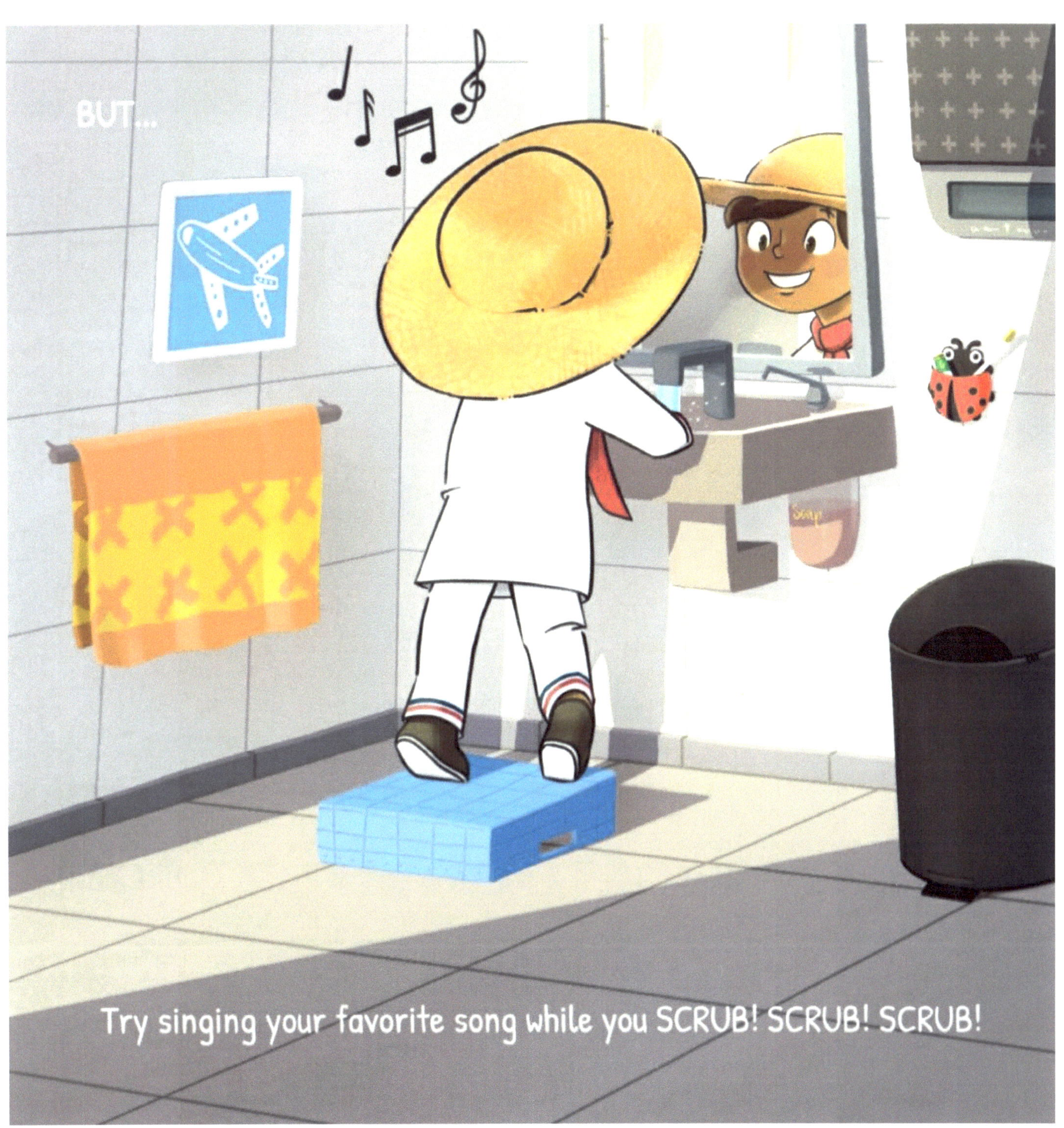

BUT...
Try singing your favorite song while you SCRUB! SCRUB! SCRUB!

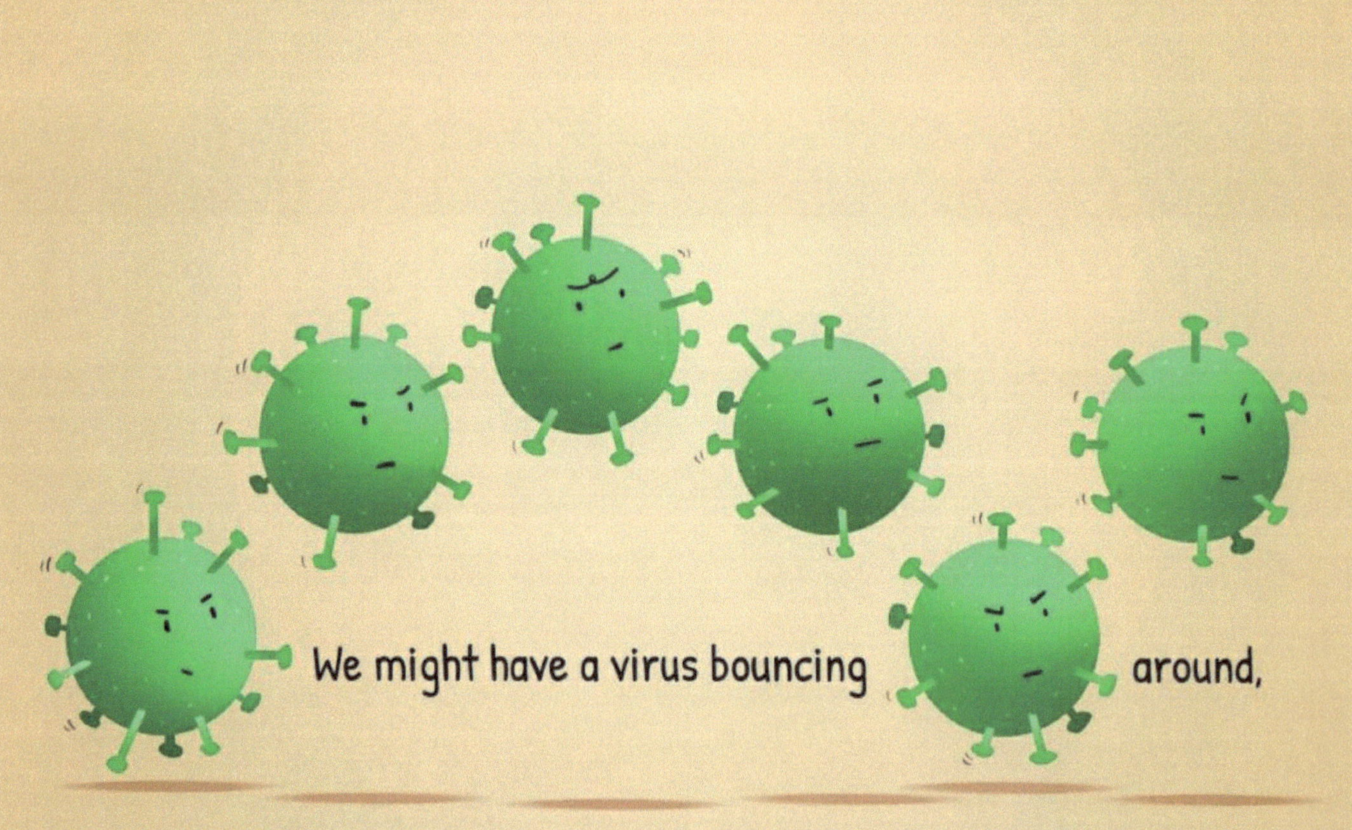
We might have a virus bouncing around,

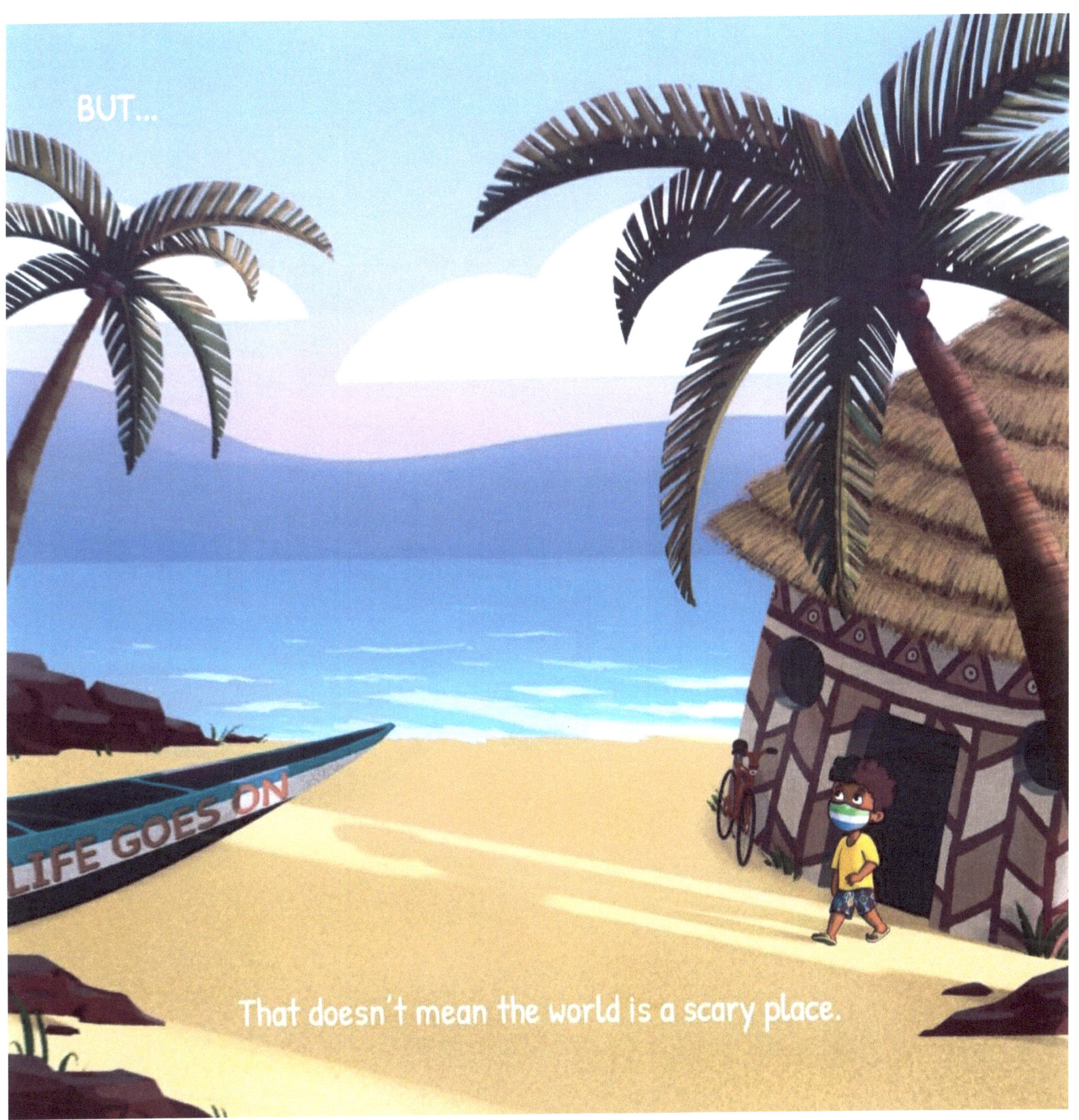
BUT...
LIFE GOES ON
That doesn't mean the world is a scary place.

Pick a book,

Draw a picture,

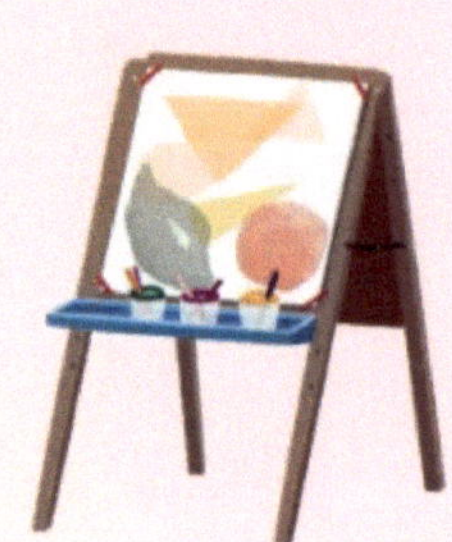

Have a dance,

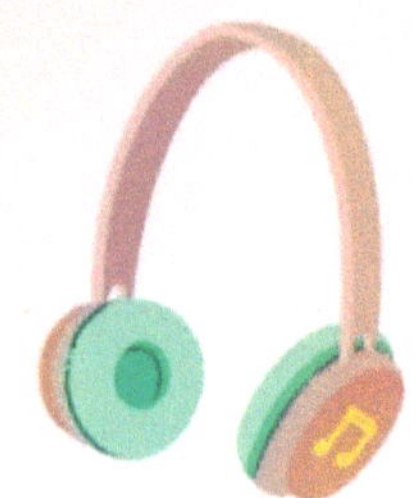

Sing a song,

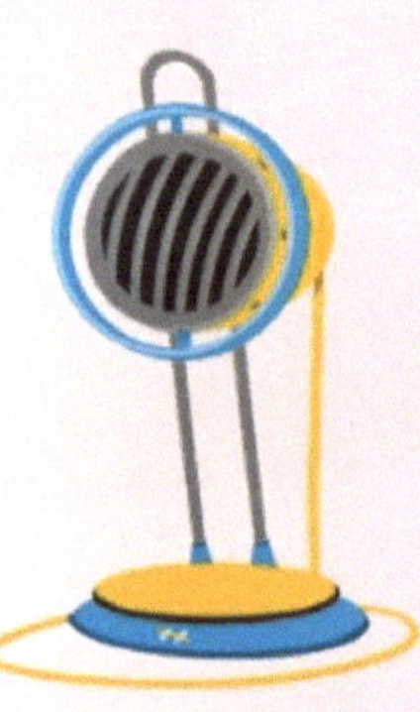

Make a fort,

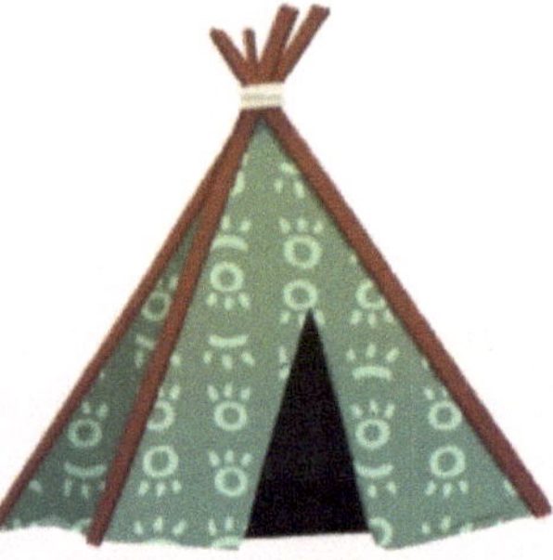

Play dress up,

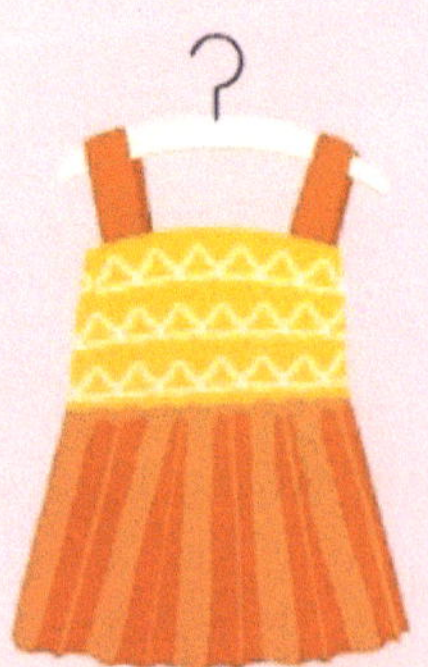

Or build anything.

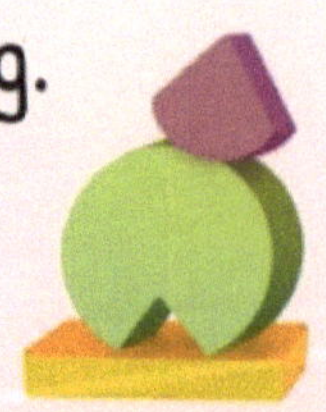

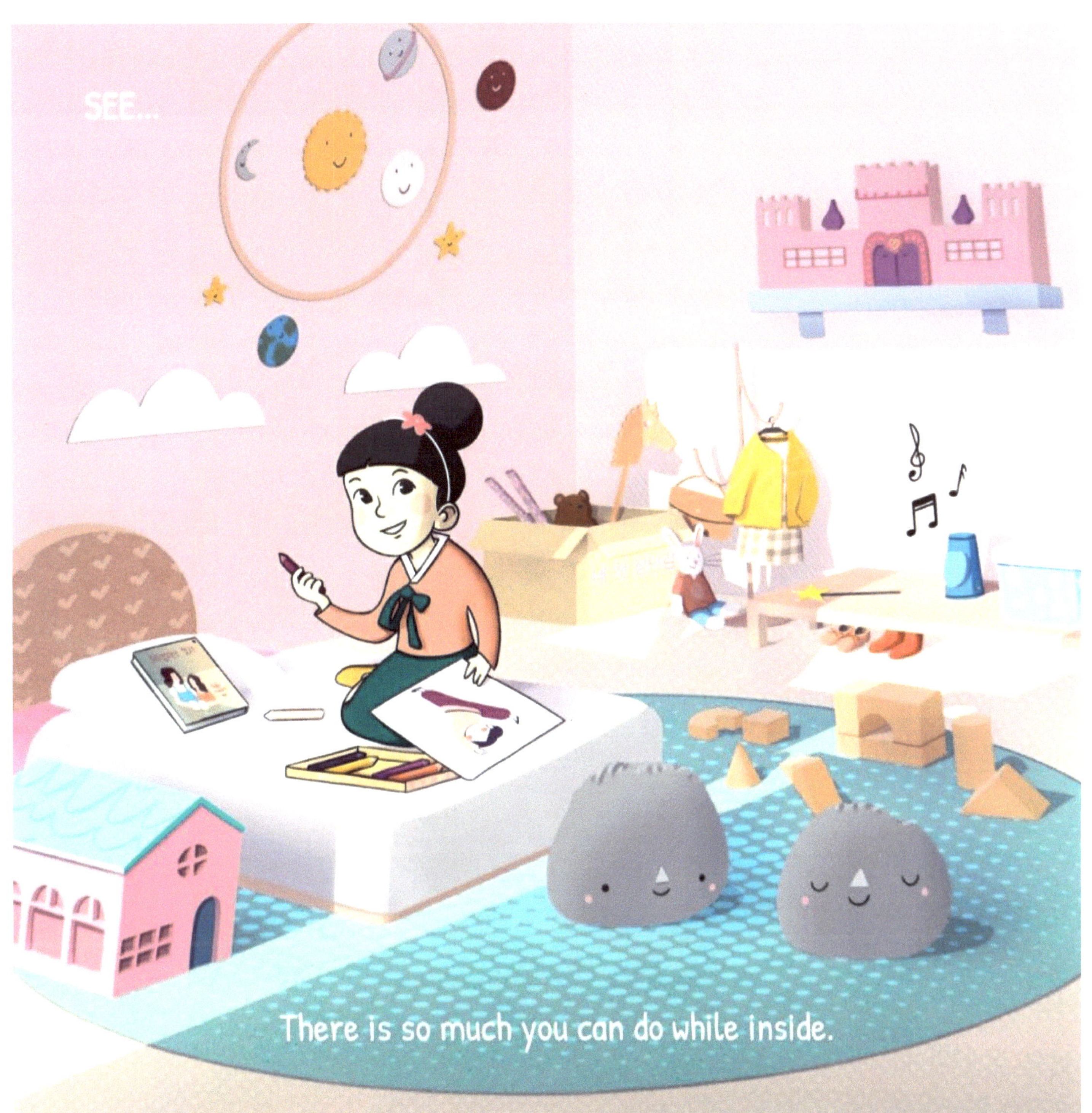

SEE...
There is so much you can do while inside.

Kumapeto

The End

समाप्त

끝

結束

Stay Safe!

La Fin

El Fin

Kraj

النَّهاية